Ultimate Guide to Knockout Lower Back Pain and Sciatica for Good

Ultimate Guide to Knockout Lower Back Pain and Sciatica for Good

(HOW PHYSICAL THERAPY CAN KEEP YOU OUT OF THE OPERATING ROOM)

Frank J. Cawley MPT

ISBN: 1533035229
ISBN 13: 9781533035226
Library of Congress Control Number: 2016911083
CreateSpace Independent Publishing Platform
North Charleston, South Carolina

"Making a difference one patient at a time."
A special thanks to all of our past and present patients, our families, friends, and of course, the entire staff at Cawley Physical Therapy & Rehabilitation for helping make all of this possible.

Foreword

This book is for all who have tried everything and given in to a life of suffering from lower back pain and sciatica: I'm here to tell you that there is hope.

In 1999, I graduated from Hahnemann University with my master's degree in physical therapy, super excited to change the world with all my newly acquired knowledge. I was ready to cure every patient that I saw. After taking my first job in a facility located in Hamilton, New Jersey, I soon discovered that the foundation PT school had provided me—although thorough—was not enabling me to produce the results I had dreamed of or imagined for my patients. Approximately 50 percent of the patients I cared for with lower back pain and sciatica had great results, but sadly, that left 50 percent of my patients who either only saw some relief, or who experienced absolutely no difference at all. I knew there had to be a better option.

In 2000, I moved back to my home town of Pittston, Pennsylvania to assist my mother and family with caring for my ill father. He passed away from pancreatic cancer just two months after I arrived. I didn't realize it at the time, but I learned a few months later that this would change my life and so many others' lives in many ways. A few months after my father's passing, I would meet the woman of my dreams—on a blind date, nonetheless—and would marry her less than two years later. We started a family, bought a new home, and somehow she convinced me to open my own private practice, all in the same year.

After many months of preparation, Cawley Physical Therapy & Rehabilitation was born in April of 2003. My success with helping patients suffering from lower back pain and sciatica continued to be good, but I was not happy with the portion of patients I was not curing or who were at a standstill with their care. The skills provided to me by physical therapy school had been tapped out. I knew I needed another way. It was not until a number of years and many hours of continuing education and training that I discovered aspects of PT that would change everything. I found ways to help my life and my patients' lives forever.

In its simplest form, the type of therapy I learned is called hands-on physical therapy. The process involves a licensed physical therapist trained in manual therapy placing their hands on a patient's body to facilitate movement of their bones and muscles to improve mobility, quickly reduce or eliminate pain, and restore function. Combined with the proper exercises for the involved area and problem, this began producing phenomenal results that far exceeded my prior successes. Patients were healing faster and with less time needed in our care.

At that point, I knew I had found the key element that was missing from my training in physical therapy school and the early years of my career. I had discovered the key form of PT care that enabled me and the staff at Cawley PT&R to help that 50 percent of patients I was hung up on. I soon eliminated the ineffective traditional PT from my practice altogether.

Patients were able to pick up their grandchildren again, or walk through the grocery store without hanging onto the cart or needing to sit down. They could sleep six hours without waking up in agony. They could go on vacations and enjoy their lives without the misery of lower back pain and sciatica.

If you fit into this category of lower back pain or sciatica sufferers, read on. I assure you that by the conclusion of this book, you will have more knowledge and information than most regarding your pain. More importantly, you will have an opportunity to take action with a specialist who is skilled in treating lower back pain and sciatica This will allow you to achieve the life-changing transformation you've been looking for. You too can become one of the thousands of patients who have been successfully cared for at Cawley Physical Therapy & Rehabilitation. This is why I wrote this book: to give each and every person out there who is suffering with lower back pain and sciatica a natural alternative to medications, injections, or surgery.

CHAPTER 1

The Role Physical Therapy Plays for the Patient

What Is a Physical Therapist?

Physical therapists are highly educated, licensed healthcare professionals who can help a patient reduce pain and improve or restore mobility. In many cases, this can be done without expensive surgery and often reduces the need for long-term use of prescription medications, eliminating potential harmful side effects.

Physical therapists are licensed by the individual states. Currently, physical therapy programs culminate in a doctorate degree in physical therapy. There are many different types of fields associated with PT that a therapist can enter upon graduation.

The expertise of a physical therapist lies in their ability to differentiate between a variety of musculoskeletal problems; they are also direct care medical providers. Direct access care is different for each state, but where available, it enables an individual to go to any physical therapist with a direct access license, for any musculoskeletal related problem, without seeing their physician first. Pennsylvania is a direct access care state.

Does a Physical Therapist Have the Proper Knowledge to Resolve My Problem?

A physical therapist's education provides them with more than sufficient knowledge and information to treat the majority of musculoskeletal related problems. Physical therapists are very skilled in treating orthopedic disorders, especially those pertaining to the spine. PTs use many different forms of treatment when caring for an individual.

Some of the items they may use include modalities that may include heat, ice, ultrasound, or electrical current. They often utilize manual therapeutic techniques that involve the therapist actively placing their hands on a patient to provide movement or increase tissue mobility and motion.

Lastly, a huge component of a physical therapist's treatment is learning the proper exercises that can help restore strength, improve mobility, and overall, return function to the patient.

Physical therapists rank in the top three medical professionals who treat spinal conditions. To date, the Cawley PT&R staff has treated upward of four to five thousand individuals suffering from lower back pain and sciatic symptoms.

How Many Patients Have This Type of Problem?

At Cawley PT&R, lower back pain (LBP) and sciatica patients make up nearly 70 percent of our annual caseload. Coincidently, nearly 70 percent of all people will suffer from LBP and/or sciatica at one point in their lifetime. Even worse, 99 percent of those people will experience relapse or chronic pain, especially if poorly treated.

On average, our office receives approximately four hundred visits per week related to lower back pain and sciatica. To date, our physical therapy team has received in excess of fifty thousand visits for lower back pain and other related spinal disorders.

What Is Your Success/Graduation Rate?

Early on in my career, my success rate was under 50 percent. After learning hands-on physical therapy combined with the proper exercise, we have increased that success rate to 80-90 percent or more.

The speed of recovery can vary based on other issues such as past medical history, prior treatment, and the time since the onset of the injury. Compliance with care is also critically important.

Do I Need to See My Doctor or Get a Prescription to Go to PT?

In the state of Pennsylvania, there is something called "direct access care" that enables a physical therapist who possesses the direct access care license to see an individual without a physician's prescription for up to thirty days.

People will often comment, "Should I see my doctor for this?" After your examination, a skilled physical therapist will be able to determine the cause and source of your problem and immediately begin treatment to remedy your problem. If there is a complication, they can refer you back to your physician immediately.

The physical therapists at Cawley PT&R are in constant communication with a patient's physician. We keep them in the loop and updated on the progress regarding their patient.

How Does a Physical Therapist Know What Is Wrong Without an X-Ray or MRI?

In most cases, a physical therapist is able to determine the cause and/or the diagnosis of your problem based on the mechanism of the injury. Patient complaints and symptoms are also very useful in this process. MRI results, although often helpful, can also be inconsistent with the actual issues or complaints that a patient has and therefore aren't always necessary.

X-rays can be valuable for determining if there are any bone issues, such as fractures or dislocations and so will be recommended if such a problem is suspected. Usually, this is easily determined based on patient factors such as age, injury, and their symptoms or complaints.

However, the bottom line is that, when a patient is improving, experiencing relief, and getting better, there's no need for testing at that time.

When Will I Know if My Physical Therapy Is Resolving my Problem?

Generally speaking, with proper care, most patients will experience relief within one or two visits. The types of questions a patient should be asking themselves include: Is my pain reducing? Is my range of motion increasing? Is my strength improving? Most importantly, is my level of function returning?

Once all of these things are accomplished, patients are provided with an updated home exercise program and graduate from their PT.

CHAPTER 2

What Does Successful Care and Complete Relief Consist of?

What Will My Treatment Consist of, and How Many Visits Do I Need?

At the conclusion of your evaluation, a skilled physical therapist will be able to determine the necessary time required and number of visits needed to resolve your issue, as well as what your treatment will consist of.

Generally speaking, depending on the number of body parts being treated and the area involved, average treatment time for each session is roughly sixty to eighty minutes. This can depend on multiple factors, including the severity of the symptoms and the response to treatment.

What Is Hands-On PT?

Hands-on physical therapy can come in many forms. One is something called a "mobilization," which is when a physical therapist places their hands on an individual and applies force to produce a movement or increased mobility. At Cawley Physical therapy and Rehab, mobilization is the most used hands-on method and generates the greatest improvements and benefits. A vast majority of PT clinics do not use this skill set, and patients are truly missing out.**

Another form of hands-on PT is stretching. Stretching can be done in many ways, but the ultimate goal is to improve the overall mobility and elasticity of the tissue being stretched.

Traction is also a form of hands-on therapy. As it pertains to the spine, this describes how we may use a moderate amount of force to create a separation between the joint surfaces of your spine to reduce pressure and pain.

Isometric exercises can be used as well. These strengthen without movement.

Finally, massage (or myofascial release) is a very common form of hands-on PT that is used to reduce pain, improve tissue elasticity, and restore function

**How Is Hands-On PT Different or Better Than Other PT?

Hands-on PT gets joints moving and improves mobility, which helps reduce pain quickly, and in certain cases, provides instant relief. It works by reducing compressive forces and presents little risk for the majority of patients.

In addition to non-invasive physical therapy, each patient also receives direct one-on-one contact with their therapist, as well as a consult, every time they enter the clinic.

Lastly, hands-on PT will set the foundation that enables individuals to exercise with greater ease and movement.

Will I Need to Exercise? If So, What Type?

Yes, every individual needs to and should exercise. The type of exercise prescribed is commonly based on which of the three common causes of low back pain or sciatica the patient has.

My fellow clinicians and I frequently hear comments to the effect that "I am too old to exercise." This is false! Clinical studies have been performed on individuals up to ninety-five years of age that have shown strength and mobility improvements through proper exercise. The most important thing that strengthening does is to help increase stability and reduce the future risk for further injury or harm. Resistive exercise also helps to strengthen and improve bone density.

Will I Need to Do These Exercises for the Rest of My Life?

Exercise is good for both young and old and should be incorporated into each individual's daily routine. It is a good idea to perform the specific exercises learned in physical therapy several times a week, and they can be performed indefinitely. The variety of exercises we teach can and should be periodically updated.

At our clinic, we never discharge a patient: We graduate our patients and establish a re-visit appointment for two months after the day of their last visit. This follow-up keeps an open loop that allows the patient continuous ongoing interaction with a physical therapist in the event of a flare-up or a new problem.

Additionally, other forms of exercise can be very advantageous, such as walking, biking, yoga, or even meditation; all have extreme benefits.

Can PT Help Me Avoid Injections or Surgery?

Physical therapy can eliminate the pain from common symptoms of diagnoses such as stenosis, herniated disc, osteoarthritis, and sacroiliac dysfunction. Physical therapy enables people to naturally reduce pain and inflammation.

At the same time, exercise can help release bodily chemicals that aid in natural pain relief. When the proper exercises are performed in conjunction with hands-on physical therapy, there will be a rapid reduction in lower back pain and sciatica, further eliminating the necessity for injections or surgery.

After My Pain Is Completely Gone, Is There a Possibility It Will Come Back? If so, Can PT Help Again?

The pain does return on some occasions. It's possible that patients could suffer a re-injury, a flare-up, or possibly even a new problem. The good thing is that you can return to PT for ongoing treatment. It is possible for an experienced practitioner to determine if the symptoms are from the same injury as before or a totally new problem.

Physical therapy can help again, but treatment may be different depending on the cause and symptoms found during the new examination. In some cases, patients with the same exact symptoms as before can be experiencing the issue due to a totally different problem.

CHAPTER 3

The Biggest Mistakes People With Lower Back Pain and Sciatica Make

Why Do People Ignore Lower Back Pain and Sciatica?

This is by far the number one biggest mistake low back pain and sciatica sufferers make. They IGNORE IT!!! Most people believe that symptoms will go away or that they'll simply get used to it. Patients we see here at the clinic will commonly mask or otherwise "put a band aid on it" in the form of a heating pad, ice, or a topical pain reliever from the grocery store. The problem with this is that it often treats the wrong area and the wrong problem.

Can Lower Back Pain or Sciatica Go Away on Its Own?

Lower back pain is complicated and there many unique diagnoses, but usually problems do not go away on their own. The longer symptoms persist, the greater the likelihood that they won't go away and that the patient's condition will in fact progressively worsen. Also, if problems continue without proper medical intervention, there is greater risk for increased harm, damage, or even permanent injury.

Even if the pain does go away, it is likely to come back, especially if the cause was not addressed properly.

When Is It Too Late to Try PT?

It is never too late to try physical therapy—but the longer you wait, the greater the likelihood for slower healing and more damage. I use this analogy: If you park a car on a hose for a second and quickly move it, the hose will be fine. If you park the car on the hose for an hour or two, it might have some form of damage. If you park the car on the hose and go on vacation for a week, the damage to the hose is probably going to be permanent and the hose may no longer be any good.

In a nutshell, the sooner to the onset of your symptoms you seek care, the greater the likelihood of decreasing and eliminating the problem. Unfortunately, PT is commonly overlooked by doctors in favor of initiating medication.

Why Doesn't Rest Take Away My Lower Back Pain or Leg Symptoms?

Rest can be beneficial for some issues or problems. However, generally speaking, movement (including hands-on physical therapy) and proper exercise is a much better option. Rest may temporarily alleviate the leg symptoms, but the actual issue is not being properly addressed. Proper positioning and posture at rest is often an important factor as well.

Can I Just Walk the Pain Off?

For certain diagnoses, walking will surely increase lower leg pain and can potentially increase lower back pain. Walking on uneven and inclined surfaces can also cause increasing pain symptoms. Short distances are okay at times, but greater distances have a likelihood of increasing your leg and lower back pain symptoms.

However, walking does have positive effects, such as increased endurance, mobility, and strength. It is also useful because it will release endorphins, providing natural pain relief.

I Am Very Busy and Don't Have Time. How Long Is Each PT Visit—and How Long Will I Be Receiving Treatment?

I tell all my patients, "You are never too busy to take care of yourself. If you don't take care of yourself, you are no good to anyone else. You only get one body and one go around in this lifetime."

Physical therapy sessions average sixty to eighty minutes, depending on how much is involved and how many areas of the body are treated. Frequency of visits start at three times a week. We then we work toward reducing that number while progressing toward graduation from PT services. A updated home exercise program is then provided.

The number of sessions each patient requires is going to depend on a number of factors, including past medical history, overall health, mechanism of injury, prior treatments, and prior surgery.

Is PT Expensive and Does My Insurance Cover It?

Compared to the cost of prolonged medication, injection, or surgery, physical therapy is very inexpensive and nearly all insurance companies provide PT coverage. Some insurance plans may have a deductible or co-pay; in some cases, insurance plans may also have coinsurance.

All of these vary depending on your plan. Some—I'd even say most—plans have visit limits for physical therapy services ranging from twenty to fifty per calendar year.

Generally speaking, PT is very reasonable and we have very flexible payment plans as well as inexpensive self-pay rates.

CHAPTER 4

What Can I Do at Home to Help With the Pain and Healing Process?

Will I Learn Home Exercises From My Physical Therapist?

On day one of treatment, patients receive exercises that they can begin performing to help with the healing process. At Cawley PT&R, each physical therapist will provide their patient with a home exercise program after the evaluation.

These home exercise programs may include routines such as stretching exercises for increased motion and mobility, or strengthening and stabilization exercises that help increase the stability and integrity of the core and legs.

The exercises can vary and may include bending positions, extending positions, or neutral positions depending on your problem and our findings upon evaluation.

There are two main types of exercises that can be performed. The first category is isometric, which is strengthening without movement; the second is isotonic, which are exercises performed through a range of movement, often utilizing some form of resistance.

Do I Need Fancy or Expensive Equipment to Perform My Home Exercise Program?

Most people can perform their exercises in the comfort of their own home, on a bed or on the floor as applicable. Body weight exercises often work the best, using the natural resistance of gravity to aid in the difficulty or ease of the exercise.

You can use ankle weights if you desire some resistance, but this is not necessary for the exercise to be effective. Affordable ankle weights are common and can be purchased at your local store; they usually range from one to five pounds.

Another option is the TheraBand, a resistant elastic tubing.

Pool exercises are often a great form of treatment as well. The pool enables an individual to decrease the weight-bearing forces normal physical exertion requires on land. Swimming is typically performed in a warm environment, which aids muscle relaxation and increases soft tissue flexibility.

Another positive benefit of the pool is that it can simultaneously be resistive and assistive. We will often utilize the indoor, in-ground pool at Cawley PT&R to initiate exercises for people with spinal problems who are very unstable or weak and who cannot tolerate the exercises on land.

What if I Don't Have a PT Table?

Not a problem: All of these exercises can be performed on the floor, bed, or sofa; in some instances, the exercises can be performed in multiple positions.

Some people will opt for a physio ball (or Swiss ball), which is an oversized ball that people can perform exercises on or use as a comfortable chair. I have seen some cases where patients have utilized a floor or yoga mat for comfort.

For example, one exercise called hip abduction can be performed while standing by moving your leg out to the side away from the other leg, and can also be performed while lying on the unaffected side and lifting the leg toward the ceiling or in the traditional way of lying flat on the back and thrusting the leg out to the side. Each of these applies a different degree of resistance based on the effect of gravity: minimal effect of gravity, maximum effect of gravity, or negligible effect of gravity respectively.

Does Posture Affect My Healing?

Posture is very important when it comes to the spine. I have found that people will affect a certain posture to alleviate the pain. Sometimes we have poor posture secondary to weakness instability; sometimes we're just plain lazy. Sitting and standing postures can vary depending on a patient's problem, symptoms, and conditions.

The majority of change to an individual's posture is due to age. There's no one I know out there who is taller at fifty compared to when they were twenty-five. This height reduction over time may range from a half an inch to several inches. This is commonly due to the degeneration of the discs in our spine as well as arthritic changes.

Should I Wear a Back Brace or Support Belt?

It is my professional opinion and recommendation that if you are in an activity or job that requires repeat heavy lifting on a regular basis, then yes, a back brace may be warranted.

For everyone else, avoid it. A back brace gives your spine and body an artificial means of support, thereby tricking it into feeling stable and strong when it is not.

In such cases, the muscles need to be strengthened. The body's core comprises the back and abdominal muscles, along with the upper leg muscles needed for power and stability.

Proper lifting technique involves the bend as well as the lift itself, and is very important. Above all, avoid repetitious twisting, lifting, and bending of the spine whenever possible.

Do I Need to Change Anything at Work or Home to Help My Lower Back Pain or Sciatica?

It is not uncommon to create workstation modifications. If a person has a sedentary job, they may have to adjust their chair, desk, or even use a footstool depending on certain factors.

I will commonly advise my patients to stand whenever and wherever possible if sitting increases their symptoms, and vice versa. I highly recommend setting a timer to remind yourself to move and change position at certain times throughout the day.

In most instances, I try to avoid asking people to purchase expensive items, but occasionally an ergonomic chair may be beneficial for an individual who needs to maintain their posture and is unable to do so naturally.

A patient's mattress at home can also be problematic. Try flipping it, rotating it every few months, or try lying on another surface. If you are creative, there are a number of inexpensive ways to accommodate uncomfortable sleep habits. I find that using a pillow between my knees or under my side or lower back is often helpful.

If I Do My Home Exercise Program and the Pain Comes Back or I Get New Pain, Can I Go Back to PT?

If patients can consistently perform a home exercise program, the likelihood of symptoms returning is greatly reduced.

Upon return, the physical therapist is going to ask: "Were you doing the exercises I gave you?" You had better be prepared to show them: Do not use the excuse, "I don't have the sheet in front of me." If you had been doing them consistently for two months, you should know them by heart.

Sometimes the physical therapist will have to dig deeper: "Did you do something different? Is it a new injury? Was there a new mechanism of injury? Are the symptoms changed? Is the pain located in a new area?"

All of these relate to the patient's behaviors: A job change, a mattress change, and a work setup change can greatly impact symptoms or problems.

Regardless of these issues, returning to physical therapy is always advised.

CHAPTER 5

What Is the Cause of My Pain?

How Did This Happen?

There are three common causes of most lower back pain. First is a herniated disc, often abbreviated by doctors or therapists as HNP. Generally, these are going to be seen in individuals thirty-five years of age or younger. Men may be slightly more affected than women, depending on the studies you read.

The mechanism of injury in such cases is typically going to be traumatic in nature. The pain is going to be worse while bending forward, and typical lifting activities will often increase the severity of back and leg pain. The lumbar section of the spine is composed of five bony vertebrae designated L1-L5. Between each level there is a structure called a disc. A disc is much like a "jelly doughnut"; the outside is fibrous or dough-like while the inside is a gel or jelly-like. The disc acts as a cushion creating space between two spinal vertebrae. When a patient is told they have a herniated disc at L4-L5, this means the disc between the spinal vertebra L4 and vertebra L5 is herniated. It is only one disc, not two. Herniated disc injury occurs most commonly between levels L4 and L5.

Approximately 70 percent of physicians believe that you can heal a herniated disc (HNP) without surgery through the use of PT and other modalities. Herniated discs are commonly diagnosed by physicians based on MRI findings. The drawback to this is that there has not been a strong correlation made in the literature between herniated disc findings on MRIs and the herniated disc being the actual source or cause of the problem.

An experienced physical therapist can determine if HNP is the cause based on the findings or your initial evaluation.

Taken together, degenerative processes like degenerative disc disease (DDD), osteoarthritis (OA), and stenosis (a fancy term for narrowing) are the second most common causes of lower back pain. These are usually common in people who are fifty or older, and typically generate the most pain during standing or walking activities. The longer these tasks are performed, the worse the pain gets.

Gender has shown no significant bearing on lumbar DDD, OA, or Stenosis diagnosis; men and women are mechanically similar. While sitting, the symptoms will be alleviated. The L4-L5 region of the lumbar lower back area is the most common area where these diagnoses have occurred. The majority of patients with these problems will feel better during bending and will experience increased pain during arching or extending backward.

Physicians will generally use X-rays to determine or confirm these particular diagnoses. By examining the results of twenty people who were fifty years of age or older, we've determined nineteen out of twenty (95 percent) of those individuals with the criteria mentioned will have positive findings on an X-ray. The correlation here with the X-ray is generally stronger than that of the MRI pertaining to a herniated disk.

The third and last common cause of lower back pain is sacroiliitis, also known as SI dysfunction. This also equally affects men and women. It is common to see associated bowel and bladder problems when this diagnosis is indicated.

Sacroiliac dysfunction is very sneaky, it can be difficult to diagnose properly, and it can be seen in patients as young as fifteen or as old as 90+. Individuals who suffer with this particular problem often have difficulty squatting or lunging. They will have trouble getting in and out of a car, rolling, or getting in and out of bed. This is a common diagnosis in runners.

This particular problem is commonly overlooked and people will pay thousands of dollars to receive incorrect treatment while the original problem goes unaddressed.

Generally, there is no diagnostic test to diagnose sacroiliac dysfunction. It is a clinical diagnosis based on the therapist or physician's findings and the patient's report of their symptoms.

To Whom Does This Happen?

As mentioned with the herniated disc, sufferers are generally thirty-five years of age or younger and the pain is traumatic in origin.

For degenerative disc disease, stenosis, and arthritis, most patients are fifty years of age or older; it is very common to diagnose these through X-ray.

Regarding SI sufferers, age varies from 15-90, men and women are equally affected and there is no diagnostic test specific to SI dysfunction. SI dysfunction is also commonly seen during or post pregnancy.

Why Am I Waking Up at Night?

This is a difficult question to answer and will require further digging to find out specifically what the issue may be. If lying down flat on the back causes increased pain, it is most likely degenerative disc disease or stenosis. Herniated discs are also known to be a source of this pain.

If movement, rolling in bed, or sleeping in a sitting position causes the pain to intensify, then sacroiliac dysfunction may be the source of the problem.

Lastly, stenosis is typically responsible if pain is caused by lying on the stomach.

These are guidelines, but when we see individuals in the clinic and they report these various symptoms in these various positions, the type of pain in each position tends to accurately correlate to their diagnosis.

Why Do I Have to Sit Down After Five to Ten Minutes?

For the most part, if patients stand or walk for longer than ten to fifteen minutes and experience increased symptoms of lower back pain and sciatica, the cause of symptoms is going to be stenosis or degenerative disc disease and arthritis.

If standing and walking result in increased lower extremity symptoms, the cause can be degenerative disc disease or a herniated disc. The diagnosis is dependent upon other symptoms as well as the history and type of mechanism of injury. It's also worth noting that if sitting and flexing (bending) of the spine decreases the pain and pressure, DDD is likely the culprit.

Why Does It Hurt to Sit for More Than Fifteen to Thirty Minutes?

The primary issue associated with sitting pain is sacroiliac dysfunction. A herniated disc can also be a cause of the problem, depending upon certain criteria. These afflictions cause worsening pain when people transition from sitting to standing positions. The same pain is encountered when getting in and out of a car or in and out of a bed, or in professions that require constant changes in position from sitting to standing and vice versa, like a car salesman.

Do I Need to Get Tests, Including X-Rays or MRIs?

In most cases, testing is not necessary. A trained and skilled physical therapist should be able to determine the proper cause and treatment necessary based on examination alone.

X-rays tend to be most helpful in determining bony issues such as fracture, arthritis, etc., while MRIs are most commonly used to diagnose soft tissue dysfunction such as disc herniation, cysts, tumors, or possibly a muscle or tendon rupture. Ultimately, the findings don't always coincide with the patient's primary complaint.

Will My Ability or Function Ever Return to Normal ?

It's highly probable that function will return and pain will decrease—if the patient follows the prescribed physical therapy treatment. Consistency with treatment and discipline in exercise is crucial. With a lifestyle that includes proper exercise, nutrition, rest, and healthy living habits, the general prognosis is for improvement.

CHAPTER 6

How Does This Pain Happen?

What Did I Do to Cause This?

Degenerative disc disease, arthritis, and stenosis are the most common causes of lower back pain requiring physical therapy for individuals 50 years of age or older. The typical causes are overuse, genetics, occupation, trauma, lifestyle, and, possibly, being overweight.

Sacroiliac dysfunction is often a traumatic mechanism of injury that can be related to a fall or damaging misstep. In women, giving birth can often lead to sacroiliac dysfunction.

Herniated discs are generally traumatic in nature.

If I Was Hurt in an Accident or a Fall When I Was Younger, Could That Cause Problems Now?

It's possible. Trauma causes inflammation; when inflammation is not addressed, it is allowed to fester and accumulate, generally with debilitating effects.

It can only get worse. Chronic inflammation causes chronic spasms, tightness, loss of motion, and will often lead to reduced strength, decreasing levels of function, and ultimately a poor quality of life.

Can a Hip, Knee, or Ankle Problem Lead to This?

Absolutely. The ankle bone is connected to the knee bone, which is connected to the hip bone which ties into the pelvis and ultimately the spine itself. Leg dysfunction can commonly lead to changes in gait and posture. All this can lead to poor ergonomics and lifting habits, which in turn can cause mechanical and structural changes; therefore, the leg problems and the symptoms of lower back pain and sciatica are all associated.

Was I Born This Way?

Hereditary factors are not usually the cause of pain. While traumatic birth can be a possible issue, it is rare. Still, some people can be born with spinal dysfunctions such as spina bifida or other complex diagnoses, which are outside the scope of this book.

Can This Just Happen for No Reason?

Depends on the cause. Herniated discs, spasms, or sacroiliac dysfunctions can develop randomly. However, degenerative disc disease, degenerative joint disease, and osteoarthritis don't just happen overnight. They are a culmination of small injuries over time.

It has been proven that a sneeze or cough—which approach speeds in excess of sixty to one hundred miles per hour—can cause a herniated disc or other issues, such as muscle spasms. Something as simple as getting in and out of a car or bed can do it. I commonly hear the proverbial complaint, "I woke up and it was there."

Unfortunately, I am a true testament to that statement. In my senior year of high school, I woke up and tried to get out of bed, but couldn't—so I know how it feels.

Is There Anything I Can Do at Work to Reduce or Prevent This?

Many things can be done at work to alleviate symptoms. Having a proper workstation setup is paramount. Positional changes should be made periodically even if an appropriate workstation is available.

In addition to active steps for improving the work environment, there are passive habits that can be fostered. Maintain proper posture, avoid repetitious behaviors, and bend and lift properly whenever possible.

There are some professions where avoiding these damaging behaviors is infeasible. It may be a drastic scenario, but changing jobs could be the only solution if the damaging behaviors can't be mitigated.

Does Eating Properly and Living With Healthy Habits Help?

Without a doubt. There are many foods that are high in natural antioxidants, free radical killers, and phytonutrients, which are very effective at combating the common causes of inflammation. Also, there are a plethora of natural brand anti-inflammatories, including Omega-3s. Foods that are high in protein help to build and maintain muscle, which is very valuable when trying to increase muscle integrity, strength, and stability. Foods that are high in vitamin B help with nervous system activity. Also, magnesium, calcium, vitamin K, and vitamin D can help with muscle and bone health.

CHAPTER 7

How Long Will My Pain Take to Go Away?

Will I Be in Pain for The Rest of My Life?

Consistently attending PT, following the physical therapist's recommendations, maintaining proper exercise, getting enough rest, and eating healthy will have dramatic impacts on a patient's prognosis. It's highly probable to regain mobility and reduce or eliminate pain if these positive lifestyle changes are followed.

What Is the Average Time itTakes in PT to Start Feeling Better?

This depends on multiple factors, including type of injury, time frame of injury, location of injury, past medical history, and prior issues.

Many patients are generally going to see significant relief with decreased pain and inflammation after the first three visits. Visits six through twelve see 75 to 85 percent restoration of motion strength and improved function.

After the twelfth visit, patients see an 80-90 or even 100 percent return to prior levels of function, pain resolution, and are able to resume life as normal. Of course, this varies for each individual, but this is a good example of the recovery timeframe based on my past experience with thousands of patients.

Will Leg Pain Take Longer to Go Away If I Also Have Lower Back Pain?

Not necessarily. The goal for people experiencing leg symptoms is to centralize the pain from the leg to the back, and then focus on eliminating the lower back pain.

For example, if someone is complaining of pain from their back radiating all the way to their foot, then we perform the hands on therapy followed by therapeutic exercises. If we can reduce those symptoms to the calf or into the back of the upper thigh after a visit or two, then we know our treatment is working.

It is good to alleviate lower back pain, but if the leg symptoms increase, it is generally not a good sign and treatment may need to be modified.

Leg symptoms (including weakness) often take longer to reduce or eliminate. Coincidentally, people with this issue have probably had the symptoms for a much longer time frame without seeking proper care.

If I Have Had Pain for Years, Will It Take Longer to Cure Than Someone Who Has Only Had It for One to Two Weeks?

Not entirely, but the idea is to treat the symptoms as soon as possible. For example, the closer we can get to taking care of someone at the onset of their pain, the greater the likelihood that improvement will be faster and last longer. When patients are treated closer to the onset, it gives the physical therapist a greater chance of reducing secondary things associated with the actual problem. Muscle spasms, poor posture, weakness, and loss of function can all be eliminated early on.

I have seen people with a twenty-year history of lower back pain and sciatica symptoms that were reduced or eliminated in just a few sessions, utilizing the hands-on treatment as well as the exercises that we have discussed.

If I Have Leg Weakness, Will It Go Away and Can I Get My Strength Back?

Leg weakness usually comes after leg pain, tingling, numbness, or burning symptoms. It is often associated with a greater duration of time than the onset of the pain or sensory changes (numb tingle burn). This is another key reason why we tell people to try to seek care sooner.

Leg problems that commonly arise may include symptoms like unequal reflexes and drop foot. Drop foot is basically a person's inability to hold their foot up while they walk, with the foot dropping down to the ground because they can't control it due to a damaged nerve. Nerve damage can also lead to bowel and bladder control issues or incontinence.

Who Can Determine How Long It Will Take to Get Better?

Physical therapists will be able to, for sure. They can establish a plan of care on day one and should discuss the treatment with you. The PT will give an approximate time frame for recovery as well as a breakdown of the stages throughout the process. A therapist may, for example, indicate that you are in the inflammatory stage as well as when you're expected to see motion and strength improvements, and finally when they feel that full function should return.

It is feasible to accomplish some goals in just a few sessions. Communication between the physical therapist and patient during each visit is paramount in this effort.

If I Have Other Medical Problems, Will I Heal Slower?

In some cases, yes. Many health concerns, such as the presence of certain medications, blood disorders, thyroid dysfunction, prior back surgery, scoliosis, cerebral palsy, multiple sclerosis, diabetes mellitus, and muscular dystrophy can impede the process of healing. This is a small sample of many medical problems that affect back pain and sciatica.

Afterword

W e have covered a variety of scenarios and how they may affect your recovery time. My hope is that reading this book has given you a better understanding of lower back pain and sciatica.

Broadly, we have a good understanding of how physical therapy helps lower back pain and sciatica, what successful care and complete relief of pain consists of, the causes of pain, and the approximate timeframe it will take for the pain to go away. For patients, we know the biggest mistakes that sufferers of lower back pain and sciatica can make, and also what they can do at home to help with the pain and healing process.

In conclusion, as my way of saying thank you for taking the time to read my book, I am offering you—or a loved one or friend—a one-time free screening for lower back pain and sciatica or related issue. All you need to do is pick up your phone and dial 570-208-2787, then tell my office that you read my book and are ready to take advantage of the free screening. The number of free screenings is going to be limited to the first 50 callers. Please do not hesitate—I would hate to see people in pain miss out on this great opportunity. I look forward to meeting and treating you in the near future.

Gratefully yours,

Frank J. Cawley

About the Author

Frank J. Cawley, MPT, received his master's degree in physical therapy from Hahnemann University in Philadelphia, Pennsylvania. He has treated more than four thousand patients for lower-back pain, sciatica, or both.

Cawley lives with the love of his life, Courtney, in Pittston, Pennsylvania. They have four children: RoseMarie, Juliet, Francis, and Beau.

www.ingramcontent.com/pod-product-compliance
Lightning Source LLC
Chambersburg PA
CBHW061937280526
45787CB00004B/1632